AF885315

Memoirs of the Divine

True golden™

By
Christopher Raingem Cookson

www.raingem.com

INFINITY
PUBLISHING

All rights reserved. No part of this book shall be reproduced or transmitted in any form or by any means, electronic, mechanical, magnetic, photographic including photocopying, recording or by any information storage and retrieval system, without prior written permission of the publisher. No patent liability is assumed with respect to the use of the information contained herein. Although every precaution has been taken in the preparation of this book, the publisher and author assume no responsibility for errors or omissions. Neither is any liability assumed for damages resulting from the use of the information contained herein.

Copyright © 2002 by Christopher Cookson

ISBN 978-0-7414-1259-1

Printed in the United States of America

Published January 2012

INFINITY PUBLISHING
1094 New DeHaven Street, Suite 100
West Conshohocken, PA 19428-2713
Toll-free (877) BUY BOOK
Local Phone (610) 941-9999
Fax (610) 941-9959
Info@buybooksontheweb.com
www.buybooksontheweb.com

Scriptures of Truth

The Tree of Humanity (Introduction)

We, humanity, have been blessed with the freedom to master the Universe, and the glory of life our Creator gave to us must never be taken for granted. Truly, we are all born upon the "Tree of Humanity", and we are all given the rights to inherit the rich blessings of the Heavenly Father and to live with great abundances. Aye, we are all living under the same sun and night facing one life and one death, and we are all purchasing the rights to live or perish forever as life and death is set before our lives. Let us all destroy the works of evil and love each other with endless mercy, fairness, comforts, and thanksgivings to our Creator so we will live a life of joy, peace, and liberty. Let us not walk in our foolish ways seeking sinful lusts, envy, hatred, jealousy, violence, drunkenness, drugs, conspiracy, sinful murder, or any other wicked deed; for by the Sword of Justice, all sins are destroyed, and every righteous person that belongs to the Heavenly Father deserves a beautiful home and a promising, fruitful life. There are enough foods in the world to feed every creature; there are enough drinks in the world to quench the thirst of every flesh; there are enough clothes in the world to comfort every being; and there is enough wood in the world to build a home for every family. Long as we live, let us never stand before the Heavenly Father as spirits who rebelled against His Infallible Throne of Truth, but as spirits who stood against the great follies of the world, and not tolerate Injustice to destroy our families and friends. That shall be our true faith in the Heavenly Father, and through Him, we, the ones who defends Truth, will succeed in everything we do for the love of His Most Holy Kingdom and humanity.

So be it.

The Spirit of Truth

Our Heavenly Father is simply ineffable. Everything changed in my life in the winter of nineteen-ninety-three when I was lost and facing tribulations impossible for any man to bear because I have been suffering from Muscular Dystrophy since I was five-years-old. For the first time in my life I searched for the Heavenly Father in spirit and truth, and I believed only He had the answers to why I am put on earth.

I remember lying in bed praying for forgiveness and deliverance. After an hour of praying, I was about to fall asleep, but then I felt the greatest feeling I ever had in decades of suffering. A warm radiant came upon me, and this warmth was full of love that no words can describe. I was in complete comfort, and visions flashed opened right before my eyes that revealed many revelations from our Heavenly Father. At first, I witnessed chaos and different shades of purple clouds surrounding me everywhere. In the far distance I saw a bright light and I came very close to it, but I never reached the end. I heard a Voice from Heaven, and the Word spoke: *Lo and behold*, I am the Spirit of Truth, Justice, and Salvation. Now that you have believed in Me, you shall bear witness to Me, and the cloud of Unholiness shall be removed from legions who love to bathe within the ocean of Sin. And verily I declare, My Eternal Love, Life, and Grace is true, and My Glory stands forever. Write everything you hear and see, and give My Truth to all you can:

I responded: Have mercy upon me for I have sinned against You, and I am tired of suffering. I want to help others when so many of my friends and family have been so kind to me and have helped me. I do not want to leave this world until I my life has been made worthwhile by doing a great deed for humanity.

He spoke: My son, truly, you are forgiven and your heart is pure before My Holiness. You have faithfully repented to be free, and by the Fire of My Hands, I have torn down the walls of Sin for you. I love you, and that is why I will grant you many seeds of Truth that shall produce boundless crops, and My reapers shall bring the harvest to Me. For truly, I am the Good Farmer, and you a good servant. You honor is to take all the seeds of righteousness I give and sow them into the holy lands of Man.

And I responded: Father, you are too kind to me. I would love to plant Your seeds for You, but what if others will not listen or what if they condemn me for telling them the truths I hear from You?

He spoke: Let the wise hear My Voice of Voices, and let the wise glorify My Love. Those who love Me hears My Most Holy Voice and I will lead all who believe in Me to My Eternal Kingdom of Life. Those who do not love Me will call upon My name on "Judgment Day", but I will be deaf to the loveless, and I will be blind to the unmerciful, for they have fallen from My Grace by walking away from My Spirit of Righteousness and Truth. And all shall see that I deliver those who love Me, and not Damnation.

I responded: Yes, Heavenly Father, I will be glad to do Your Will. Simply tell me what to say and what to do, and I will do all that needs to be done for Your sakes.

Then I saw a Hand of Fire descend before me holding a ring with three keys attached to it. One key was gold, another was silver, and the last bronze. And the Heavenly Father spoke: Take these keys and open the gates I will lead you to.

I took the keys and an old, narrow road flashed in front of me. I saw a tall wall of crystal on my right, and the ground was filled with boundless flowers, grasses, and bushes, yet, not one weed was in sight. As I walked down the narrow road I saw a large arch entrance with a bronze door. I went and opened the bronze door with the bronze key, and I saw a glorious park filled with absolute beauty. In the center stood three great trees that bloomed many colors at once, and the colors changed continuously. And the Heavenly Father spoke: Go to My Tree of Truth and pick seven red leaves and eat them as you shall have knowledge on how to please Me. Then write all seven truths I give you to feed others.

I went and did as I was told, and these are His seven red Leaves:

Let the wise worship Me in secret within the temple of your body with all your heart, soul, and mind, and I will listen to you and your prayers.

Let the wise protect all my righteous creatures as I love them, and I will keep My Glory within you.

Let the wise keep your soul under My Grace, and I will rejoice within you and celebrate My Life with you.

Let the wise teach others to love, serve, praise, worship, pray, and exalt Me, and I will hold you close to My Heart and embrace you.

Let the wise keep My Wings of Faith and Wisdom within You, and I will protect you and deliver you from all your trials.

Let the wise feed My lambs My Love and Wisdom, and I will be pleased with you, and I and My angels will dwell within you in peace.

And let the wise stay away from dead works, doctrines of men, radicals, false prophets and false priests, and I will bless you with blessings that shall never perish; for, verily I declare, I am the Glory of Life, and those who love Me shall be comforted by My Light of Love, and they shall know that I am with them throughout all their trials, and I will set them free from all sorrow and hopelessness.

After I recorded the seven Leaves, the Heavenly Father spoke: Come out of My Park and lock the door behind you.

I did as I was told, and I walked down the old road that seemed several miles. I came upon a second arch entrance with a silver door, and I took the silver key and opened the door. As I looked in, I witnessed a vineyard miles long and miles wide, and I saw a winepress near the end with a giant cave where I knew all the wine was stored. And the Heavenly Father spoke: Go find twelve red grapes that are ripe and crave them, and you shall have knowledge on the Glory of My Eternal Spirit. Then write the twelve truths I give you to all who thirst for My Spirit.

I did as I was told, and these are His twelve Red Grapes:

I am the One Who gives Grace. Those who love Me do the works of My Righteousness, and they shall have My Mercy.

I am the One Who feeds the world Truth. Those who love Me follows Me and teaches humanity My Wisdom that gives the spirit Life.

I am the One Who blesses Peace. Those who love Me are merciful as lambs, and they feed the world My Truth and Justice.

I am the One Who delivers Freedom. Those who love Me defends My Throne of Justice that destroys the works of Iniquity without hesitation.

I am the One Who pours Wisdom. Those who love Me learns from Me, and I will lead all Mine to My Cloud of Eternal Glory.

I am the One Who shines Love. Those who love Me cares for those afflicted by diseases; for even as I gave humanity the gifts of friendship, I have given the gifts of wisdom to break all slaveries.

I am the One Who destroys Sin. Those who love Me are wise to repent and keeps their temple clean from all disgrace, for when I come in secret, there is no error in sight.

I am the One Who renders Justice. Those who love Me stands up for My Truth, and those who are My warriors of faith and bravery shall live to see My Glory.

I am the One Who is the Fountain of healings. Those who love Me will be healed from all illnesses, for I have the power over all, and everything is possible through Me.

I am the One Who grants Eternal Life. Those who love Me believes in My Begotten Son, the Messiah who took away the sins of the world, and those who do the works that are pleasing to Me shall have eternal life.

I am the One Who is Salvation. Those who love Me cry to Me for deliverance, and I shall set all who believe in Me free forever.

I am the One Who Is, Who Is to come, and Who is Eternal. Those who truly love Me have set their faith and hope upon Me, and I am their Foundation of Strength as I bring all My beloveds into My Eternal Kingdom of Peace and Glory.

After I recorded the twelve Red Grapes, the Heavenly Father spoke: Go find twenty-two white grapes that are ripe, and crave them as you shall have knowledge on more truths, then write the twenty-two truths I give you.

I did as I was told, and these are His twenty-two White Grapes:

Behold, all false prophets and preachers who preach the doctrine of men and not Mine are walking in the tunnel of darkness. Turn to Me quickly and walk in My Light before you lose your life forever.

All religious leaders who are only after the money and power instead of following Me, behold: I do not know you, and I do not show My mercy upon you. I am the Passover Lamb, and those who love Me and believe in Me shall be cleansed from their sins, and they shall never see death as I will give all My faithful ones eternal life.

All religious leaders who offer up prayers for the people and withhold them from praying to Me themselves listen: I am not deaf, and I know the hearts of All. Let My children worship My Spirit in Truth, and let My faithful ones pray to Me in secret within their own spirit; for truly I declare, I will guide all who love Me, and I will give My endless love and comfort to all who mourn to be free.

All who confess their sins to priests and not Me listen: I am the Light of Salvation, and if anyone wants to be free, come to Me and I will lead you to My Path of Righteousness; for verily I declare, only I have power over all sins, and only I have the keys to set you free.

All religious leaders who claim that I bless by tithes listen: Truly I declare, I do not bless by tithes. Those who place their faith in Me and do My Righteousness shall be blessed; and if anyone wants salvation, come to Me, and I will give you My Grace and you shall have eternal treasures.

All who love to rape, kidnap, murder, or commit suicidal bombs listen: I know your crimes and no one escapes My Wrath. My Justice is coming to slay the wicked, and My Truth is coming to put away evil forever. And behold, this is the solemn truth: each day throughout humanity, My Sword has slain countless who love the darkness more than My Light.

All who love to bathe in fornication, adultery, incest, or any other immoral sexual sin are bathing in the Fire of My Wrath. Stop sinning against Me, and come to Me and bathe in My Light of Love forever; for verily I declare, if you come to Me in peace, I will be your Beloved Father and I will lead you all along the Path of Righteousness that will set you free from all shame.

All physics, mediums, and wizards who love to lie, rob, and deceive multitudes listen: Why are you deceiving My creations by your vain works? Return to Me and behold the Glory of My Holiness that gives the world Life; for verily I declare, not one devil will succeed in getting into My Eternal Kingdom of Love, Justice, and Liberty where evil is cast out forever.

All religions who refuse to worship My Holiness in spirit and truth by worshipping carnal ordinances have been deceived by the Evil One. Let the wise worship Me Who is the Living and the Truth. Those who love Me do the works that are living, not dead.

All who love the life of a cult listen: Come to Me and I will give you My Ceaseless Love and Joy, and you will not be judged with eternal damnation.

All who love to buy and sell from the Evil One are seeking to be slain by My Sword of Truth. Come and eat My Bread of Life that I have given to all without charge and you shall never see death, for I have given this Sacred Gift to all who set their hopes upon My Glory so they may be delivered from eternal damnation.

All who love the ways of communism are bound to suffer the eternal lake of fire prepared for the Unloving. Where is your mercy, and why do you use the forces of Slavery against the ones I have created? I demand you, the ones who hate, oppress, steal, and murder, to love all humanity as I love them, for I do NOT know Evil. Countries who do not surrender from communism shall face My Wrath, and behold, the powers of Communism shall fall, for I will set liberty to the poor and the oppressed, and the slaveries of the world shall perish forever.

All who love to worship false religions and false gods are walking away from My Holy Kingdom to suffer poverty in the heart. Let your heart not be deceived, for only I am Eternal, and only I am Supreme above all as I created all. Let My faithful ones come to Me, and I will be your Foundation of Strength; for verily I declare, those who believe in Me are protected under My Wings of Glory forever.

All leaders in governments or religions who love to cheat, lie, and deceive citizens for their own immoral pleasures shall receive My Wrath. Why has Satan deceived you, and why have you betrayed Me by your disgraceful works? Repent, and fall under My Grace now, for My Sword of Justice is coming to put away the wicked who do not love their neighbors.

All who love to deceive, hate, abuse, conspire, or follow any other immoral works have their souls hooked to the Anchor of Sin. If you have ears to listen, understand: I am the Way, the Truth, and the Life, and I am the Throne of Eternal Justice. If anyone wants to be free, come to Me and I will take you off the Hook that is cast to the Dead Sea.

All who fail to love the poor, disabled, elderly, children, women, men, mammals, and animals are falling off My Tree of Life where rotten fruits are tossed to the eternal fire. Come to Me and surrender from your hatred, and I will keep you in My Eternal Kingdom of Life and love you as My own child forever.

All who cannot be merciful and hate evil shall not receive My Mercy, for I demand you, the ones who hate, to be merciful and loving to all. I am the Light, and you the seed. When the clouds of Sin engulfs you, you cannot live without Me.

All who hate and refuse to love their neighbors shall see My Wrath of Justice. The Spirit of My Holiness is Truth and Justice. I am the Father, and you the children. When the Thief steals you from Me, the thorns of Sin chokes out the flowers from your soul-garden, and it is too late.

All who love to follow the traditions of men and not My Ways are not pleasing Me. Those who love Me and seek to please Me do the works that are living, and My Light floods their holy temples always.

All who love Evil, why perish with the ashes? Let your heart not die, and come to Me so I may give you eternal life. I demand those who believe in Me to love My Righteousness always. Those who love Me will cast down all wicked deeds and imaginations and live within My Light of Truth forever.

All who do not follow My Light and Love, why be a slave? For verily I declare, I came into the world to take away the sins of the world so those who seek My Most Holy Grace and Love shall have hope and everlasting glory.

All who love to appear into My Holy Churches as a devil dressed into an angel of light, why burn down the temple of your soul? Woe to you who deceive My creations to worship the One without love or mercy. Those who love Me will sin no more and worship Me in spirit and truth always, for I am the Good Shepherd, and I lead all My lambs to My Kingdom where Sin is nevermore.

Truly, I declare to all. On Judgment Day, those who refused to repent and fall under My Grace shall be eliminated from My Book of Salvation, and they shall not receive eternal life. Take heart and listen, for I have warned you. I am Truth that delivers Justice to all, and those who are wise, fear Me and sin no more.

After I recorded His twenty-two White Grapes, the Heavenly Father spoke: Come out of My Vineyard and lock the door behind you.

I did as I was told, and I continued to walk down the narrow road, and after some time, I came upon a third arch entrance with a golden door. I took the golden key and opened the door. As I looked in, I witnessed a divine garden with boundless trees, streams, flowers, grasses, etc. And the Heavenly Father spoke: Go find twelve red cherries on My Tree of Faith and crave them, and you shall have knowledge on My blessings. Then write My blessings to feed others eternal hope and joy.

I did as I was told, and these are His twelve Red Cherries:

Blessed are the ones who loves Me, for glory shall be theirs.

Blessed are the ones who believes in Me, for the gifts of eternal life shall be given to them.

Blessed are the ones who listens to Me, for they shall see the Truth.

Blessed are the ones who trusts Me, for they shall be secured.

Blessed are the ones who feeds My lambs wisdom, for they have fed Me.

Blessed are the ones who gives drinks to My children, for they have given Me sweet drinks.

Blessed are the ones who follows Me, for they shall be delivered from Sin and Death.

Blessed are the ones who cannot look upon sin, for they are My beloveds.

Blessed are the ones who come to Me faithfully for My Grace, for I shall have mercy upon them.

And blessed are the ones who endure faithful and loving to Me, for they shall be loved and welcomed in My Glorious Kingdom forever.

After I recorded His twelve Red Cherries, the Heavenly Father spoke: Go find twelve oranges on My Tree of Justice and crave them, and you shall have knowledge on more of My blessings, then write My blessings.

I did as I was told, and these are His twelve oranges:

Blessed are those who loves and follows Me, for they are My beloveds that worships Me in Spirit and Truth.

Blessed are those who destroys evil, for they are My true lambs following My Righteousness all along the path of Justice.

Blessed are those who fears Me and does no harm to the innocents, for they are My true children enjoying eternal life in My Most Holy Kingdom.

Blessed are those who gives hope to My orphans, for they are My faithful ones.

Blessed are those who cares for the elderly, for they are My heart of peace.

Blessed are those who helps the disabled, for they are My heart of mercy.

Blessed are those who inspires the poor, for they are My heart of hope.

Blessed are those who loves their family, for they are My heart of kindness.

Blessed are those who comforts their spouses, for they are My heart of love.

Blessed are those who does no harm to children, for they are My heart of beauty.

Blessed are those who love animals, for they are My heart of joy.

And blessed are those who feed themselves My offerings, for they are My heart of life.

After I recorded His twelve Oranges, the Heaven Father spoke: Go and find seven rare golden apples on My Tree of Salvation and crave them, and you shall have more knowledge on My Truth.

I found the seven golden apples and craved them, and these are His Truths:

If anyone wants to live, live by My Love and worship Me in Spirit and Truth.

If anyone wants to be free, come to Me and receive My Grace.

If anyone wants to be just, let Me show you the Way that leads to eternal life.

If anyone wants to be loved, let Me be the First and Last Love of your life.

If anyone wants to hear the Truth, listen to My words and not the Unholy nor those who worship Unholiness.

If anyone wants peace, learn by My Wisdom.

And if anyone wants eternal life, come to Me, for I Am Hope, and I am the Key of Glory given to all who believe in Me.

After I recorded His seven Golden Apples, the Heavenly Father spoke: Come out of My Garden and lock the door behind you.

I locked the door, and the old road vanished before me as I was brought back to the bright light and the purple clouds glowing within the chaos. Then I spoke: O Heavenly Father, You are the Way, the Truth, and the Life! Shall I write anything else?

Then He spoke: Love of Mine, verily I declare, you have swallowed thousands of seeds and you shall sow them into the holy lands where good soil is produced, and all good crops grown by the Light of My Holiness will be given to Me when the harvest is due. Then all My crops will be brought to me and I will give all the blessings I have prepared for those who faithfully follow Me, and I will welcome all of you into My eternal Kingdom where the lambs and shepherds live in peace with the wolves and lions.

I responded: You are too kind and merciful. Anything else you want me to record for Your sakes?

And He responded: Let all who hear My Most Holy Voice, listen, and sin no more; for truly I declare, I am Truth, I am Justice, and I am Salvation as the Sword of My Holiness destroys the works of evil forever. And behold, My Justice in which never falls, My Liberty is forever. Let My lambs come to Me, the Eternal Shepherd, and I will give you hope and rest from the wolves, for no one can live without Me.

And I spoke: If it is not too much to ask, how much longer must the world suffer diseases?

He responded: On My Tree of Life hangs a sacred fruit that will heal all illnesses. When it is time, I will send an Archangel to bring it to the world, and all shall eat its bitterness and be free, and I shall be pleased.

I spoke: If I may ask, when will this happen?

He responded: That is a mystery sealed within Me.

Then for a brief time, His Spirit left my heart at joy and wonders.

Proverbs

O Heavenly Father, all creations shall forever exalt Your Holiness beaming Everlasting Liberty and Grace from the Light of Your Majestic Spirit. You are the Spirit of Glory that cannot cease from blooming Truth, and You are the Root of Holiness that cannot be uprooted by hands of Ire and Malice. And when the shadows of darkness dare to bring the armies of soul-slayers before Your Throne of Justice, the Mighty Wrath of Your Holiness shakes the foundation of the heavens as the Holy Fire from Your breath roars and no spirit can stand and not tremble, for You are the Glory of Righteousness that conquers all wars of Folly, and You are the Warrior of Justice that triumphs all battles of Injustice.

All Glory to You, Heavenly Father, Your Most Divine Spirit leads the children of Peace to Your Loving Kingdom where the powers of Sin cannot enter. Your Glory protects our sacred spirits built with the Temple of Your Justice, and Your Holiness manifested upon us breaks the iron chains of Slavery. And truly, Your True Vengeance destroys the shadows of Sin that roams across the earth night and day seeking its prey to imprison and devour its temple built of clay and water.

All exaltation to You Heavenly Father, for the seeds of wisdom You have stocked in my dawnlit-temple. I exalt You forever, for Your light is the Most Holy Fire that is the Word of Truth, the Breath of Holiness, and the Light of Life. All seeds we sow today, Your Righteousness shall lead the spirits who cry for mercy to the Fountain of Life, and when they drink from You, the sins shall be stripped from their naked spirits, and they shall be clothed in robes of liberty. And tomorrow they will not be cold and abandoned, nor imprisoned to the birdcage of Shame. They shall be where You are in peace, and they shall witness the Divine Power of Your Immortal Glory sitting upon the Most Holy Throne with the Everlasting Laws of Justice in the Left Hand, and the Everlasting Covenant of Life in the Right Hand. So be it.

On The Heavenly Father

O Heavenly Father, You are the Most Holy Spirit, Truth, Justice, Salvation, Mercy, Wisdom, Faith, Love, Joy, Peace, Life, and Liberty. All exaltation belongs to You forever.

Heavenly Father, You are the Archetype of all creations. Who can even begin to contemplate Your Most Holy Existence? I am so honored to follow You, and I shall do all that pleases You.

Heavenly Father, You are the Spirit of spirits, Light of lights, Unit of units, Body of bodies, and Creator of creations. I shall trust in You, and I shall do nothing but love You with the spirit of my soul that feeds You fruits of joy.

Heavenly Father, You are the ineffable Cloud filled with Everlasting Love and Glory. I follow You through the desert of trials, and never shall I leave Your guidance that leads me to the pastures of eternal life and liberty.

Heavenly Father, I am one swimming within the Violets of Your Heart, like a man in joy without the shadow of death clinged to my soul; and I peacefully swim the waves of eternal life, as I am free to float upon the ripples of Justice rolling to the shore without a shame.

Heavenly Father, the earth is not my refuge for You are my Refuge. For why behold sands of sins in my heart when they smuggle the Flame of Your Glory that ascended me to life?

Heavenly Father, because of You, I am freed, loved, and blessed. Thank You for everything you did for me each passing day, for I shall do all you ask me to do and please You. You are my Eternal Heavenly Father of Truth.

Yea Heavenly Father, I am disabled and I give sacrifices every moment to glorify You. I am like a cloud fabricated with the light of dawn, but the dead cannot see my beauty that shines upon the world.

The Heavenly Father is coming to all of us to bring His Justice. Let everyone fall under His grace before it is too late. For if we refuse to repent and turn from our sins, the gates of Hell are opened to us upon Judgment Day. But if we are wise and not be ignorant to His Voice, we shall find pastures of peace where sin cannot enter.

The Heavenly Father's name is not "God." The word 'god' derives from the pagans. Simply put, our Creator never gave us its name. Our Creator told Moses "I am that I am."

Our Heavenly Father is not human. Our Creator is a Divine Spirit that created both male and female, therefore, our Creator has the spirits of both sexes.

Heavenly Father, You loved the world so much You came and died for our sins. Only Your Divine Spirit would sacrifice such a Glorious Love. It is like watching a child grow for a brief time, and then as You became a Man, You died before our eyes. And as You ascended, Your Perfection shines and the cold storms fade forever.

Heavenly Father, You are a Great Tree that bears good fruit. First, Your Sacred Seed is sowed in my soil, then Your Divine Roots grow strong and wild, and then Your Perfection grows out of my ground tall and beautiful as the child of I runs towards Your Glory with ceaseless joy.

Heavenly Father, You come to all races and revealed Yourself to those who love You. Those who claim You only reveal Yourself to one race has fallen into the Pit where hogs wrestle in the mud of Folly.

Only You, Heavenly Father, knows when the end of the world will be. No man will ever know the year, month, day, hour, minute, or second. We are but children who cannot tell time when sands of the Hourglass never falls upon our command.

Heavenly Father, You are the Creator of all seeds of Truth. No matter what religion, old or new, if a religion bears witness to a truth, then it is from Your Spirit.

Heavenly Father, one that denies the existence of Your Glory denies the existence of their beauty.

Heavenly Father, a righteous child is Your best delight, for the child is celebrated with the angels of Your Kingdom and they all dance and sing together.

Heavenly Father, I sacrificed my foolish deeds and exchange them in for great fruits from Your Garden, and I became a seed of Holiness, a root of Strength, and a flower of Beauty.

Heavenly Father, I am a solitary son working in the distant fields of rapture to stock up wheat for Eternity.

Heavenly Father, it is painful for a babe to come forth from the womb of its mother. Surely, how much more suffering will cost us to come forth from the womb of the earth? Whatever the pain must be, we must face it.

Heavenly Father. Let those who are lambs of Your soul visit the sick, poor, prisoner without a heart of pity, but rather with arms of Mercy, and lights of wisdom.

The sun chases the coldness of the earth, yet You, Heavenly Father, love me as I confide in You. For truly, who can live without the Rays of Your Truth that beams from the center of Your Most Holy Spirit?

Yea Heavenly Father, Your water purifies my spirit. For I believed in You, and as I drink from You, I became as wells of living water, and multitudes come to gather for a refreshing drink of life.

Yea Heavenly Father, You decorated the space with absolute beauty. Let the beautiful ones also decorated their soul in the name of Your Love.

Heavenly Father, Your Divine Will is everything pure in desires. Who can wear the face of Shame forever when the mask does not have to be there?

Let the wise do the will of our Creator all times for a great reward in heaven. One will seek its Silver, then its Gold, and then its Diamonds.

Heavenly Father, let the wise worship You every moment. For truly, who can't realize its soul alone is either a church of Your Holiness, or a church of Satan?

Loving is the one who is afraid to sin, for they know if they did, they'd break the heart of the Heavenly Father. For who would want to do harm to the One who created all the heavens and the earth, and who would want to put a sword into His Heart knowing He created our beauty? Let us be the creatures of Justice, and let us be the hands of mercy and caring.

Humbled is the one who lives for the glory of the Heavenly Father, for they are warriors of Faith as they never fear death.

We are put on earth to learn, yet to be tested. Every moment, people die and are being separated to eternal life or eternal death.

True is the one who prays in secret, for that's where the Heavenly Father lives in discreet.

Patient is the one who waits for freedom from the Heavenly Father.

To be holy is to be loved by the Heavenly Father, and to be foolish is to be crowned by the Foe. Yea, the Heavenly Father loves those who choose to be blessed by Life.

My friends, the Heavenly Father lives in your very soul, and He is constantly waiting for you to seek Him so you will know Him. There is no reason for you to not go to Him and behold His Love.

The Heavenly Father wants you to know His Grace so you will live with Him always in peace and joy. Seek it, hold it, cherish it, and embrace it.

If you are poor and live in the ghettos, honor it and stay holy for the Heavenly Father will bless you rich.

Life on earth is easy to get away with crime, but they will never succeed on Judgment Day when they stand before the Heavenly Father. Behold, the slain of Justice are many.

Verily, if you walked into the Kingdom of the Heavenly Father, you will not see any divisions. In Heaven there is nothing but everlasting love and friendship from all creatures and they all worship their only Creator.

The greatest price one can pay is a cross assigned by the Heavenly Father, for it buys the gifts of eternal treasures.

One who hides their sins is like a dog hiding their bones; but the Heavenly Father always remembers where the bones are hidden.

One who allows Truth to be silent is a thief, but one who reveals the truth is a man of Justice.

One of the greatest gifts the Heavenly Father gave Man is the power to choose, but holy are those who loves Righteousness. They are like roses without a thorn, and their beauty is perfected by the rays of the Sun.

Loving the loveless is acting like sons and daughters of the Heavenly Father. Who can feel good turning away from those who want to be loved?

Zeal the Glory of the Heavenly Father righteously and you shall see Him face to face.

One that leaves everything for the Kingdom of Heaven is the best servant of the Heavenly Father. Such servants are rare gems scarce to be found.

True is the one that beholds the wisdom of the Heavenly Father.

True is the one that eats out of the garden of the Heavenly Father.

Lambs lay down their lives for a sacrifice. Peaceful are those who fade for the love of the Heavenly Father.

One that gives everything for the sake of the Heavenly Father shall have treasures beyond measure.

The flesh is weak. Serve the Heavenly Father with all your spirit.

One who is racist against humanity is far from the Heavenly Father. Peaceful are those who love their neighbors.

One who is wise and humbled pleases the Spirit of the Heavenly Father.

Justice is only perfect with the Heavenly Father's wisdom. Without it, the world is dead.

The love of the Heavenly Father knocks upon your door constantly. True are those who open the door with joy.

The Heavenly Father gave Man the breath of life, how could one stand to forsake Him and His kingdom? Repent and sin nevermore.

To walk toward the light of the Heavenly Father is wonderful, but to bathe in the love of the Heavenly Father is divine.

The Heavenly Father gave Man the breath of life. The least we can do is honor Him.

Gold is rare to be found, but so is the Heavenly Father that is your very Creator. Therefore, which is greater to behold?

One who washes their soul more than their clothes is indeed great to the Heavenly Father.

One who does not sin grows like a great apple tree, and multitudes of the Heavenly Father come to taste its sweet apples.

One who sacrifices their life for the honor of Truth shall rest in the Kingdom of the Heavenly Father.

To be book smart alone does not please the Heavenly Father; but to be living righteously pleases Him very much.

One who sows the seeds of Man with the knowledge of Truth is great in the Heart of the Heavenly Father.

On The Messiah

The Messiah is the Heavenly Father who destroyed all illnesses upon the cross He died on. The hour is coming when all who belong to Him and suffer this moment shall be free forever and never will they be forced to drink a cup of poison again.

The Messiah was not born on December 25. December 25th is the birth of a sun god. There simply is not one scripture in the New Testament that says our Savior was born on December 25th.

The Messiah destroyed the works that are dead upon his cross and He made alive the spiritual works that are living.

The Messiah is the Final Sacrifice for our sins, and the animals that were sacrificed before Him symbolically represented Him. There is absolutely no justice in sacrificing anymore animals when the Messiah put an end to dead offerings. We now offer things that are living.

Our sins forsook The Messiah and nailed Him to the cross. Because of our iniquity, we hated Him and failed Him. Let us not forsake Him anymore by surrendering our follies so He may have mercy upon us.

Truly, The Messiah was the Lamb without blemish that was slaughtered and laid on the Brazen Altar of our Sin Sacrifice, and after He stripped off the flesh, His Spirit resurrected from the grounds like an Eternal Tree of Life bearing many different sacred fruits. And forever, we may eat His spiritual fruits to live in peace.

Those who fear The Messiah shall cast down all wicked imaginations. For even as a lumberjack chops down trees, so must man chop down Unholiness.

Those who believe in the Messiah shall not baptize with water, or perform foot washing, or perform suppers, or any other dead work. One who truly believes in the Messiah must have faith in Him, and do the works that are living, not dead.

Those who believe in the Messiah beholds His Spirit, for they have the glory of the Holy Spirit that teaches them the ways of the Heavenly Father.
Which is greater, the churches or the Messiah? If you get cast out of churches because you refuse to follow dead works, be grateful for the Messiah will be honored of you for following Him.

Those who seek the Messiah shall be fulfilled in spirit.

To believe in the Messiah is to bury the carnal and resurrect spiritual.

When the Messiah never surrendered to temptation on the cross or before, surely one can overcome fear, pain, diseases, loneliness, and death with Him.

Even as the black holes grave the stars, the Messiah graved the old carnal ordinances by fulfilling the scriptures that testified of Him.

The Messiah is the Sabbath. The Sabbath Day has been fulfilled on the cross that the Messiah died on. The Messiah is rest for your souls. Go to Him whenever you feel you need rest, and He will give you rest for His burdens are light.

The Messiah is the Spirit of Comfort. Without Him, no one is comforted.

The Messiah sent the Holy Spirit to teach us the truths so we may follow Him and be Holy with Him.

Truly, those who do the dead works of Satan is against the Messiah, for you cannot serve the dead and the living at the same time.

Those who thirst for the Messiah shall receive everlasting springs of comfort.

The sun bathes the face of the universe. How much more is the Son of the Heavenly Father willing to please you?

The Messiah fulfilled all the scriptures that testified of Him. All carnal ordinances are buried upon His death, and on His resurrection, all spiritual principalities of the Messiah resurrect those who believe in Him to eternal life.

The Passover has been fulfilled by the Messiah. The Messiah is the Passover Lamb that was sacrificed upon His cross for our sins, and through faith in Him, we pass from death to eternal life. Because of Him, we are delivered from all wickedness and death.

The Feast of Unleavened Bread has been fulfilled by the Messiah. This Festival symbolized the True Bread that descended from heaven. The Messiah is the Bread of Life, and those who eat from Him shall never perish.

The Feast of First Fruits has been fulfilled by the Messiah. The Messiah is the Firstborn of all creations, and truly, He is the Vine and we are His branches that bear good fruits. Through Him, and no other, we become fruitful and live a wonderful life without wickedness in our spirits.

The Feast of Weeks has been fulfilled by the Messiah. Fifty days after His death, the outpouring of the Holy Spirit began, and we became a part of His wheat harvest. Without the Holy Spirit living within ourselves, our souls are forever dead in its grave and we never resurrect to life.

The Feast of Trumpets has been fulfilled by the Messiah. The Messiah is the Trumpet of Holiness that evil fears. If you believe in the Messiah, take His trumpet and blow loud and hard for Justice, and you shall see a new life begins and hope is established by faith in Him. Those who believe in the Messiah declares war on the wickedness in themselves and defeats all sins through His Power. Without the Trumpet of the Messiah, there is no hope, and without Him there is no life nor peace.

The Day of Atonement has been fulfilled by the Messiah. The Messiah is the one who atoned our sins upon the cross He died on, and if we believe in Him, our debts are stamped out forever by His Grace.

The Feast of Tabernacles has been fulfilled by the Messiah. After the Messiah resurrected to life, the Messiah poured out the Holy Spirit on Pentecost to harvest the souls that belong to Him.

On Grace

To fall under Grace one must surrender its old nature of sin. Sin is like an addiction of alcohol. When we acknowledge we have a problem we go in for counseling to clean up our act. Same thing with sin. We go to the Messiah to learn how to overcome our problems then we become free and fall under grace. We cannot receive grace if we are slaves of Sin.

Come into the Light by your faith and see the glory of Grace, for you shall behold a true life.

Cast down every wicked imagination that comes to your mind with the faith of the Messiah that gives grace, for you are worth more than death.

Come and see the beauty of Grace that glows eternal rainbows. You will feel a thousand times better than what you can ever imagine.

It is true. If one lacks sin, you cannot enter the Kingdom of Heaven. One must bring in the sword of Truth and destroy all sins within the spirit and fall under His grace.

It is true. If you are in the light and behold seeds of sin in your palm, you will not enter heaven. All sins must be removed. Therefore, the grace of the Messiah will help you overcome your darkness.

Surrender to Grace, and you shall be given knowledge on how to clean your soul.

Surrender to Grace, and Love will hear you.

If one takes away freedom from another, that thief shall have no grace.

If one works with terrorism, grace shall not be given. Turn away from the darkness!

If one abuses women, children, or animals, grace shall not be given. Turn away from the darkness!

Those who claim we sin everyday is a sinner who does indeed sin everyday. Not everyone sins each day, for there are angels out there who love Truth with all their souls. Even babies do not sin. To repent is to remove deeds of sin through the grace of Love.

If one wants grace, one must have faith to wash away their sins through the blood of the Messiah.

Grace is the Flower of flowers. So beautiful, so merciful, and so perfect.

Grace is the light of Salvation that shines for the universe to see. All one must do is walk out of their dark temple and believe it is there by faith.

Come, my beloveds. Come and take an eternal home by inheriting grace and walking into the light of Truth. If you look, you shall see, and if you see, you shall behold its glory.

To behold grace is to bury your old nature and put on the spirit of Truth.

We are to be pure in the soul like the Spirit of Spirits. Without this purity, souls are unclean and cast into the darkness where sin reigns. Let the true ones wash their sins away in the Blood of the Lamb, then they shall no longer desire to sin and they shall be free forever. Such mercy is the Grace of Salvation.

On Politics

A mouse lives to steal Man's food; but when the government acts likewise, they are in danger of Judgment. For verily, what profit is there is behold the deeds of Theft? True governments eats from the bread of Liberty.

Capitalism is the true way to follow and live by, not socialism or communism. Simply put, capitalism is a moral system that sets the people free from slaveries while socialism and communism created oceans of dead bodies.

Money itself does not cause corruption. It is the people who abuse it foolishly that causes corruptions.

The more the government sets the people free, the higher, faster, and perfected the nation will bloom to be.

Capitalism is the light of freedom in the world of economics. Without this light, the darkness comes with the damned and chokes out prosperity from the people. Clear, simple, and plain.

A strong nation builds a divine military to protect its country from evil. The stronger the military, the more safer we are. The more power of military, the faster we can wipe out those who defend evil.

Woe to the governments that creates more laws and less freedom, for more laws only puts the people under the chains of Slavery.

Woe to the governments that tolerate injustice for your system is unjust.

Woe to the governments that steals from the people, for you will be held accountable for your crimes!

Woe to the governments who lies to the people, for you will be held accountable for your follies!

Woe to the governments who oppresses their people, for you will be held accountable for your disgrace!

A true government is fair to the people, for such is the mercy of our Creator.

A true government destroys the works of evil.

A true government sets the people free from ALL slaveries.

Those who are in government only for the money and power shall suffer the wrath of Truth. Be aware, the Sword of Truth is coming to slay the wicked, and the slain is countless.

Tyrants, dictators, radicals are all cowards bound to suffer or suffered the Sword of Justice, and there will be no mercy when the dead refuse to be merciful and fair.

Anyone who thinks more government solves our problems is not wise. More government only creates slavery, poverty, and death for the citizens.

Justice is only perfect through our Creator. We must follow Him in order to lead a nation of Truth and Liberty for all humanity.

True is the leader who is holy, for such a man beholds a patch of strawberries without poison, and the angels eat and rejoice in its sweetness.

A true leader is great in wisdom serving all races righteously.

A true leader forbids cheating for popularity.

A true leader never defends injustice.

A true leader is not a whoremonger.

A true nation unites as One under Truth and follows the road of capitalism that leads to life.

Soon, the world will all be reigned by capitalism for the Heavenly Creator gave its freedom to us, and His Will shall be done on earth.

A true leader plants seeds in the heart of Man that grows a great cedar tree of Truth; then the fowls will come and build a nest within.

A true leader sacrifices their lives for the love of others.

A true leader must set the people free and give them hope, peace, and justice. Without justice, hope, and freedom, slavery reigns and death comes with the clouds of Darkness.

A true leader sees to it that all citizens become educated regardless of what religion, sex, age, disability, or race. Intelligence is divine, and every human being should feel the glory of its power.

O nations of the world, when will you become friends and love each other with ceaseless mercy? Let there be light in all that you do so the air will be silent from the cries of sorrow and disgrace.

O nations of the world, let there be friendship and brotherhood with all nations, for verily, we are all born upon the "Tree of Humanity". Sadly, some must fall from its tree and perish.

A nation that loves injustice will always lead a kingdom of Folly. Great are the nations where Love, Justice, and Freedom reigns.

On Crowns

Crowned is the one that is put in prison for the devil to test and not surrender their soul to the Foe. Those who brave the tests of Courage are warriors of Faith and Justice, and nothing can overcome their light.

Crowned is the one who confesses their sins and repents to the Creator of creations, for He shall have mercy upon such a repenter.

Crowned is the one who honors the ways of the Heavenly Father.

Crowned is the one who is great in faith, for the wings of the Heavenly Father shall protect and deliver them.

Crowned is the one who lives for the Kingdom of Heaven.

Crowned is the one who lives to love others, for the Heavenly Father shall exalt them.

Great are those who believes in the Messiah, for the crown of glory settles upon them.

The ladder to Heaven if far in distance. Crowned is the one reaches the clouds of Perfection.

Crowned is the one who forbids sinning, for they are seeds of beauty that blooms perfection.

Crowned is the one who is no longer under the curse of the Heavenly Father.

Crowned is the one who walks in the light of Truth and never looks back to turn into a pillar of salt.

I don't see the Messiah wearing a crown upon His head like hypocritical religious leaders. True men and women don't need crowns to proclaim their greatness.

On Marriage

Dear husband and wife, let both of you always be faithful to each other and let love seal your souls together to become unbreakable. Let there be trust and beauty, and let there be peace always as the dawn in true bloom.

To the fathers: be good to your children and never use the hands of Satan to harm your children. The Spirit of the Heavenly Father is mercy.

To the mothers: love your children and never mistreat them for if you harm them, your follies are shown to the Heavenly Father.

A newborn baby has a pure soul. Beautiful are the parents who keep it clean and merry.

Parents who teach their children to live righteously truly does care for their spirits.

Let love between husband and wife endure in faithfulness, for this is eating the sacred fruits.

If the wings of marriage are broken, try and heal the wings the best you can. If the wings are hopeless, then it is best to let it perish.

An angel cannot live under the roof with a devil, nor can a devil deal with an angel.

True marriage is built with a strong foundation. The hurricanes come, but the house endures.

Marriage without trust can never stand as a strong cedar. The tree becomes chopped down.

If the deeds of Unholiness are living with a family, cast out the wickedness before the family crumbles to nothingness.

If your child becomes disabled in any way, do not be ashamed of its defect. You would be amazed what the Heavenly Father gives to those who are brave and beautiful inside.

The book on how to raise a child is to love them and teach them wisdom.

Without mercy, a marriage is bound to crash.

Without love, a marriage is better off dead.

If Satan tries to come into your marriage, slam the door upon him before he destroys your temple.

The wings of the Heavenly Father will always protect a true marriage, and nothing can touch its sacredness for the two lovers are followers of His light.

On Work

A carpenter learns to build homes for a paycheck. Surely how much more is the Heavenly Father willing to give for living righteously? Let every spirit rise the beauty of their temple to perfection so the Heavenly Father shall be pleased, and let every soul be built with the Word of Truth so they may never perish.

A farmer of the Heavenly Father plants seeds of Truth throughout the universe, and when the fruits have been craved by the multitudes, the Heavenly Father is pleased.

A gardener plants seeds of flowers upon the land; yet blessed are the one's that bloom in the name of the True Beauty.

We must always do the works that are living, for this leads us to a world of liberty and peace.

Holy are the one's humbling themselves and work for the Immortal Spirit, for they are like a glorious spirit full of light, full of love.

One that refuses to work will lose their life, which is not wise. Come and work for the Heavenly Father and you shall receive many blessings.

The greatest job of all is working for the Kingdom of Salvation.

Work is only good if we work for the service of goodness. If we work for the sinful companies, we serve Satan.

O women who work at strip joints. Let your heart not work with Satan for he is only using you to destroy you and men by hooking you to his ire hook and casting you to the deep seas of shame and death.

If we love Truth we will destroy the works of evil to protect our families and friends. For what good are we when we hold the weeds of sin and not the wings of life?

One cannot work for the Master of Sin and the Master of Life at the same time. One is either for the Truth or against it.

True workers are the ones who are fair and just.

True workers are not lazy nor full of excuses not to work.

True workers are the ones who destroys the works of Iniquity.

On Wisdom

Wisdom is greater than Folly for Folly doesn't teach how to live. Let the wise behold the seeds of Wisdom and let the faithful sow the seeds in all the world. For when their spirit rises under the rays of Truth, they shall see the beauty that remains.

Aye, seeds of wisdom are sowed and harvested upon the soils of the followers of Truth; and the Farmer of Life patiently waits to reap the crops to bring into His Stock house.

The strongest man physically can never break a piece of iron, but the wisest man of wisdom can split the world in half.

How is it technology has increased, but wisdom to live has decreased? Cast down wickedness and receive life.

To be wise is to climb the mountain of the Heavenly Father; but to be foolish is to fall down the staircase to eternal nothingness.

Wisdom is like the wind. You cannot see it, but if you behold it you can blow away your enemies.

Without wisdom, a man is dead.

Without wisdom, a man is deceived.

Without wisdom, a man is lost.

Wisdom is infinite in knowledge and good imaginations.

Wisdom is the fruit of understandings. If one starves to death due to lack of wisdom, it is too late.

When you behold wisdom, you cannot hold foolishness in the same hand when wisdom and folly do not mix.

Wisdom is a seed of liberty. When you plant wisdom in your soul, a new life begins. But wisdom without faith to grow will never see the sunlight, nor will its bud bloom to life.

The greatest house one can build is the temple in their soul. Wise is the one that creates a castle of Holiness.

Without wisdom, a world cannot live in peace.

Without wisdom, a world cannot see the Truth.

To wear the robe of Wisdom is to be warm in the cold.

Wisdom is like a caterpillar. When one grows in wisdom, the skin comes off and butterfly wings are born to sail a new world.

To be wise is to testify the Truth.

To behold wisdom is to find beauty and life within yourself.

Wisdom is sacred. Care for it and do not forsake it.

Wisdom is a sword that devours anything wicked. Use it with the faith of Holiness and you shall conquer your tribulations.

On Truth

Truly, truth is the Spirit of Life.

Truth is the Wine of sweetness.

Truth is the Sword of Justice.

Truth is the Color of Liberty.

Truth is the Vine of life.

Truth is the Sun of light.

Truth is the Moon of peace.

Truth is the Heart of freedom.

Truth is the Seed that conquers all wickedness.

Truth is the Sacred Fruit that the faithful eat with joy and praise.

Truth is the High Mountain of perfection.

Without Truth, a nation cannot see the light of Glory, nor can the nation rise to see the light of Liberty.

Without Truth, a nation has suffered the cup of shame.

Without Truth, a man cannot rise for he is clouded with Sin.

If one wants to live, one must bear witness to the Truth.

If one wants freedom, one must defend Truth.

If one wants victory, one must follow Truth.

If the lambs of the Heavenly Father do not lay down their lives to defend Truth, how will the hungry ever be fed?

Rise in good habits, bad habits will wilt and die.

Without Mercy the world darkens, freezes, and perishes to nothingness.

The gift of Truth is richer than the world.

Even as the fall must bring death, so much the Spring bring life.

Even as the winter must bury, the seeds must resurrect.

The great one is merciful, yet not tolerate evil.

Love is perfectly known, yet sin is always shown.

Hail comes to destroy nature. I say bring hail into your soul and pound the wicked off your territory! This is a truth in a bombshell.

Without imprisonments Freedom reigns, but what happened to trust in the world that cries for Justice? Woe to those who oppress the people!

Without Peace lives misery.

If one runs into a prostitute be their friend, not their sex-slave.

To be perfect is to be pure in the soul.

The winter brings snowflakes to give nature rest. Bring winter into your soul and freeze Sin!

Flowers never beheld the seeds of Folly, and they are the beauty of Truth.

Truth is the rainbow of Peace. Each color shines the seven ways of Perfection.

Keep the key of Truth in your hand always and you shall open the Sacred Door that leads to Justice.

If you can see the Sun of Truth, you shall rise from the grounds and enfold the pedals of your flower with endless liberty.

Without Truth, the air is poisoned.

With Truth, you can conquer the world.

With Truth, you can capture Sin and overthrow Him.

With Truth, a star shines as bright as the sun and gives warmth to the world.

One who eats to relieve their anger is bound to great trouble. Be strong inside and you shall be free.

One who ignores the spirits of wickedness shall be dressed in glory.

The greatest key is the key to heaven. All one must do is to search for it, hold it, and keep it.

It is the truth; Truth is the sweet reign that rains upon those who love life.

Heaven lives in everyone's soul, but how many can shut out hell at all times? Repent, and sin no more I pray.

If all religion can't come together and unite with Truth, arguments will always be created.

If you want to get high, get high on giving and you shall see many wonders.

One burden of a disease is the measure of carrying a dozen iron tanks.

One that lives for gambling is willing to lose all they have, including their soul. Gamble no more.

One who is eager for the end of the world truly does not care for the souls dying. We need more workers to bring others to their salvation.

There are two kinds of rich people: the ones who are fair and generous, and the ones who are greedy and thoughtless towards humanity. The true rich ones are the spirits of life.

There are two types of poor people: the ones who refuse to work, and the ones fighting for their freedom. Those who fight for their lives will always find life.

One who loves to drink liquor believes they are free, but truly, they are dying inside of their souls. Seek help before you drown in great sorrow.

The greatest key one can behold is the key that opens the gates to heaven.

Rainbows shine forth its glory for all Man to witness. Man that is a child of Truth also glows for the world to behold.

Scientist everywhere searches for life's explanation, but they are lost and blind without knowing Truth first.

The best friend one could have is one that guides them out of a cold storm with their lighthouse.

It's better to pay a price for your sins here on earth rather than lose your soul on Judgment Day.

It's greater to be shy and humbled rather than being loud and proud.

The moon is lonely all life, but when Man came to land upon him, he waits for a friend to visit again. Therefore, visit those who are lonely so that that may have a piece of love to crave.

The path of destruction lies before all feet, yet great is the one who ignores its trail.

How is it those who rarely cry cannot heed to the cries of the children all year around? Comfort the cries of the children, for one day you may suffer the way they are forced to suffer.

Feed the hungry, for it is a righteous deed to do, but do not only feed them food, but feed them wisdom so they can find work to be self-sufficient.

If you love, follow, and worship the Truth, freedom will always be crowned upon your heart, and all the powers of darkness cannot take that glory from you.

On Folly

Folly is asking the holy to perform miracles to believe; but speaking Truth is the greatest miracle of all. For verily, the wise sees the signs of the Spirit when its Love reveals the glory of His name to them.

Folly is to be a free loader, but the holy lives to be loved by working and serving.

Folly is a gang of violence. Turn away from such disgrace and live in peace.

Folly is drive-by shootings. They shall one day answer to Justice for their foolishness.

Folly are the false healers who deceive for money, and behold, the gates of Sin are opened freely to them while Heaven has locked them out.

It is easy for folly to steal, but hard for the holy to be disrespectful.

It is easy for folly to hate, but hard for the holy to sin.

It is easy for folly to sin, but hard for the righteous to be holy.

It is folly not to love and care for those in prison. Truly, not everyone behind bars belongs there, and not everyone in the society belongs free. The day of Judgment is coming to all of us, and the holy are not judged.

It is folly to serve Sin and perish. Love has so much to offer.

It is folly to lead people into false religions for the grave has been opened.

It is folly to use a false tongue and cuss, for such is what Sin is made of.

It is folly to follow man-made traditions for it leads humans to the pit of Folly.

Why wear the gold of Folly when you can wear the glory of Peace?

Why dig for the diamonds of greed when you can dig for the Kingdom of Truth?

Who can stand to sin and be a slave to Sin? To think Sin has glory to offer is folly.

On Glorious Spirits

Glorious are the ones who pray in secret, for the Heavenly Father shall comfort their weariness within the solitude. For even as a baby mourns to be cared for, the hands of Love comes with joy to remove the sorrow one beholds.

Glorious are the ones who bring in the Ark of the Covenant into their soul and worship His Holiness always, for the Cloud of the Heavenly Father shall descend and dwell within them in peace.

Glorious are the ones who give praises to the Heavenly Father forever, for this offering is a precious gift from our souls.

Glorious are the ones who give thanksgivings to the Heavenly Father forever, for this is the sacrifice from our hearts.

Glorious are the ones who give glory to the Heavenly Father, for this is the meat of our spirits.

Glorious are the ones who give love to the Heavenly Father, for this is the fruit of our souls.

Glorious are those who carry the cross of sickness fearlessly, for they shall soon be free.

Glorious are those who lays down their life for the love of others, for they shall have heavenly rewards.

Glorious is the one who brings the Heavenly Father a basket full of good bread that has the taste of good faith.

Glorious is the one who is never ashamed of Truth for the Heavenly Father will always deliver them to peace.

Glorious is the one who keeps the light on within the temple of their soul. This seals the darkness out of their lives.

The stairway to heaven is far in distance. Glorious are those who run for the golden light of Truth.

Glorious are the rich in spirit for they are sons and daughters of Mercy.

An ocean of goodness lies in the Heart of Holiness. Glorious are the ones who drinks from it.

The dawn in the sky shines its beauty for the world to witness. Glorious is the one that glows their love for all.

Flesh is nothing without a spirit. Glorious are those who shine bright in righteousness and love.

Everyone can sin; it's the seed available to eat. Glorious are those who plant flowers of mercy in their soul and do not sin.

On Religion

All religious leaders have absolutely no power over souls, for every human being can worship the Heavenly Father in Spirit and Truth wherever they wander.

To be a high priest has nothing to do with the clothes one wears, or the sacraments, or the crowns, or the gold. To be a high priest, one must be able to bring justice, love, beauty, truth, peace, grace, and liberty into the world. That is what makes one a man.

Don't think your existence is just a soul, spirit, and body. You are a temple of Holiness. Everyone can worship the Creator from within. Let His Light shine, and you shall be at complete peace.

The Aaronite priesthood is no longer in effect when the Messiah buried the carnal ordinances on His death at His cross. Now all who believe in the Messiah has full access to the Heavenly Father from within their own hearts. Thank goodness for the Messiah for taking away the Key of Knowledge from the greedy and thoughtless and giving it to ALL!

Those who follow the tradition of Holy Eucharist are deceived, for the Messiah never said to make this tradition. Bread and wine does not give us life, but the Blood of the Lamb that paid our sins delivers us.

Any preacher who believes traditional ceremonies and rituals saves our souls or pleases the Heavenly Father is deceived, and therefore, deceives others with him. For truly, our bodies are a temple and we are a church of either the Heavenly Father or Satan. We can now worship the Heavenly Father in spirit and truth within ourselves always, and we have full access to His Spirit.

Preachers who thinks they are above everybody is in grave error. For truly, many who are wise shall be ashamed, and the Truth will be given to those who humble themselves before Truth.

It's easy for a preacher to claim to be a servant of Truth, but how many take the time to identify their fruits?

Listen to the Messiah. He says to pray in secret and not in public. Those who pray to the Creator in secret will be rewarded if your intentions are true.

Woe to the religions who make laws not to marry! You are not holier by restraining from sex. One is holier by doing the will of Truth and overcoming the works of evil.

Woe to those who worships stones, walls, gods, gold, or anything else dead, for they have no life. To find our Creator, look in your very soul that is a temple.

Woe to the religions who charges a fee to join their church.

Only an evil religion seeks miracles to declare humans a saint. True saints don't need men to crown them saints, but true saints seek to please our Creator by doing righteousness.

There are religions today who still try to withhold the key of knowledge from men. Woe to you who are selfish! Everyone shall have full access to the Truth, now and forever.

Woe to the priests who rape, for you shall answer to the Creator for your disgrace!

Woe to the priests who performs false healings or giving the false Holy Spirit. Behold, the Wrath of Justice comes to put away the dead.

Woe to the priests who tries to buy off their victims for sinning against them. Behold, Justice is right around the corner.

Woe to the religious leaders who use the peoples money to buy rich lawyers in order to escape your crimes. Behold, you will give accounts to the One Above, and you cannot escape His wrath!

Any religion that demands one to sign a contract in order to join a church is false.

All religions are made by one Creator, and all religions are created equal as our Creator does not put one religion higher than the other.

If you seek guidance in times of trouble, look in your soul and find your very Creator. Listen, and you will be guided. Follow, and you will be delivered. Do not be afraid, and you will be free.

Religious temples built by hands of men will crumble to dust easily by hurricanes, earthquakes; but the temples I build within souls of humanity shall never fall nor perish, nor can all the powers of darkness touch you for you are protected by the Light of Above. I am a carpenter, and I learn from the Messiah, and together we please our Creator.

If a priest loves and yet deceives people, he is false. Turn from the darkness lest the darkness defeats you.

If a priest does not know how to find, love, or worship the Heavenly Father, he is false. Let the wise stay away from such shame.

If a priest withholds the Truth from men he is false.

If a priest receives glory from men, but not from the Heavenly Father he is false.

The Holy Spirit is not about yapping the mouth off nor jumping around like a firecracker in ones butt, nor passing out like one has been struck by gas. The Holy Spirit is a teacher, and very few receive it. To receive this gift, one must be true and faithful, and one must love. When one receives the Holy Spirit, one becomes full of wisdom and truth.

A proud preacher's words lives to steal for himself, but a humble preacher lives to catch souls for the Good Fisherman within its net.

Anyone who says the Messiah is not the Heavenly Father Himself does not know the Heavenly Father. The Messiah is the Heavenly Father that descended from heaven to deliver us from Sin through His death and resurrection.

Any priest who claims the Messiah is not equal with the Heavenly Father is deceived. The Heavenly Father, the Messiah, and the Holy Spirit are the three states of Life. They are not greater or lesser than one another..they are all equal working in one Spirit.

A preacher should be wise to guide the lost soul to the Heavenly Father and Son.

A preacher who commits fornication with children is an absolute disgrace to the Heavenly Father!

There are different rankings of priests: The high priests are full of love, wisdom and truth. The low priests are babies beginning to grow and are on their way to perfection. Then you have the false priests that are after the money, power, and hold fast man-made traditions and laws.

The greatest communion is with the Heavenly Father. Beautiful are the ones who go to Him for guidance and comfort.

Great are those who received grace from the Heavenly Father.

Great are those who do everything in their power to deliver truth and justice into the world. I mean All truth and All justice.

Great are those who follows the Heavenly Father always.

Great are those who do everything they can to set souls free and end evil.

Great are those who cannot commit any kind of sin.

True are those who do not get paid to visit people.

True are those who do not follow the traditions of men, but follow the Spirit of Truth.

True are those who preach Truth and nothing but Truth.

True are those who do everything with the power of the Heavenly Father to cast down the wickedness of Satan and his sinful servants.

The day is coming when all humanity will no longer need churches to receive salvation. Salvation comes from within, and each and every one of us who are the sons and daughter of Life are a church of holiness with our bodies.

On Satan and Death

Anyone can follow Satan to hell; but great is the one that denies sinning for they shall live to see Life. For verily, the gates to hell is where sin perishes, but the gates of life is where the holy lives forever.

If we behold the seeds of Sin, we are slaves of Sin and will die in shame. Let us not behold these false seeds in which kills our spirits.

Sin is the Bread of Damnation. Those who eat this bread with merriness have died and become buried with the dirt of Shame. Eat this bread no more, and try the Bread of Life when you will feel free from all sins.

Satan causes countless to worship the things that are dead, and countless perish with him. Let your heart not be deceived, for time is running out for all of us. Let us all stay in the Light so we never perish.

Evil is Satan's sword; mercy blows away its folly.

Woe to those who teach their children to become suicidal bombers! It is better that you were never born.

Satan does everything he can to change the times and laws of the Heavenly Father. Let us not be deceived.

One that lies is one that is guided by the footsteps of Satan. Look at the footsteps of the Heavenly Father instead, and you shall see true life.

Sin feels good for the followers of Satan, but they will change their minds in hell and it will be too late. Sin no more.

Sin is a deadly disease. We must walk in the light day and night, and we must not be deceived and keep our faith in Truth. It is possible to be sinless, but it can only be done through our faith in the Heavenly Father and the Messiah. The question remains, do we truly want to be free? If so, why then do we sin again? Let us sin no more and destroy the works of evil.

Without the light of Truth, all humanity will be buried in the pits of Satan.

Sin belongs to the doomed, yet life belongs to the sweet fruits of Kingdom Come.

Peace is in the palm of Man's hand. Great is the one that keeps it safe from Satan.

The ice forms its foundation to trick all that may walk upon it. Beware of the Fool that is cold and damning to put you to sleep!

The shadow of the Fool is constantly following your footsteps. Great are those who refuse to look at Sin.

Why slave for Satan that forbids your creation when you can work for the Heavenly Father and be loved?

Death pleases the sinner, but life honors the righteous.

When sinful lusts comes to sight, shut out its presence before the Fool tricks you to fall in its tar pit.

A thief at night is paying Satan a ticket to lose their soul.

The greatest power Satan has is time. Let the Fool never win your soul to rape.

Satan always kisses you with a peck of betrayal, but holy are those who rebuke him.

Satan gave Man the right to die, but the Heavenly Father gave Man the glory to live.

Satan has slaves that hate him, but the Heavenly Father has legions of angels that love Him.

Satan never sleeps. He is constantly looking to destroy everything the Heavenly Father created.

Satan only has a little time left before his kingdom is destroyed. Until then, let the beautiful ones stay away from sinning.

One who betrays is one who kisses the feet of Satan. Betray no more.

The greatest lie the Fool can tell you is that you cannot overcome him. We can overcome him through faith in the Messiah.

On Love

Anyone can give big to its own family, but beautiful are the ones giving vast to those families of the world who have little or nothing.

How is it those who are strong rarely lend a hand to the weak? Help those who cannot help themselves.

To save souls has everything to do with love.

Love is a flame that never ceases. It gives warmth to the world.

Love is a hand of Mercy. Those who behold this hand cares for others.

Love is resurrecting the flowers of Love.

Love is the Lighthouse that guides the ships of Life home.

Love is the Bridge that lets its beloveds walk into the Land of Salvation.

Love is the kiss of a man, woman, and child that loves each other.

Love is the Cloud of Glory. Nothing can shake its Foundation for Love reigns over all.

Love is the gift of Peace. Through Love, we receive peace in spirit.

Without love, we fall into the ocean of despair and drown.

Without love, we fail in everything we do.

When love comes we should never take it for granted.

Love overcomes all illnesses.

Love is teaching others the way to Freedom.

Without love, the world sins, falls, and perishes.

One who does not love animals does not love the Creator of creations.

If love is not known, death will be lived.

The greatest love ever told and known is Truth.

The humbled one is full of love, mercy, and compassion.

Caring for the helpless is indeed an angel from Heaven.

Anyone can sin for it's the seed available to plant. Yet everyone can also love which is the Greatest Spirit that never forsakes.

When love is little in the world, death is easy to come by. Yet mankind can bring heavenly peace by destroying the works of evil.

On Peace

Peace will never be unless the works of evil are destroyed.

Peace will never be long as terrorists are tolerated to kill the innocents. We must wipe this disgrace off from the face of the earth now and always.

Total peace will never be on earth for there will always be evil or those who worship evil. This is why it is so important to reduce evil as much as possible. The more we reduce evil, the more goodness rises. Clear, simple, and plain as that one deed.

We cannot make deals with terrorists with a piece of paper. That is like trying to trust Satan, a liar, hater, and murderer. The only deal we make with terrorists is to cast them out of the earth like flashes of lightning.

Let us be the faithful servants of Peace that sows the seeds of Truth so we will bear good fruits for our neighbors to eat.

Let us be the cloud and the rain so we will give drinks of Peace to the world thirsty for Justice.

Let us be the sun and the light to give Liberty to the earth. And the light knows no darkness!

Let us be the fire that gives warmth to the world, and the fire of Truth tolerates no evil to hurt innocent people.

Let us follow Justice so we shall behold Peace.

Peace is the Foundation of Strength.

Peace is the Cloud of Freedom.

Peace is the rainbow of the Most Holy Spirit that glows its perfection across the world.

Peace are the children rejoicing together.

Before the eyes of Peace are opened, the spirit must come out of the Womb of Liberty.

We can either behold the Jewel of Peace or toss it to the sea. I kept it in my deathless soul.

Peace belongs to the souls worthy of rest. For the labors they slaved in faithfulness to Truth, the Hands of Grace and Salvation blesses them.

Peace belongs to the ones who starve for such mercy, for theirs is the life given to them.

Peace belongs to the children at heart who beseeched for glory and good health and friends, for such creatures shall behold that Sacred blessing.

Peace comes by the Sword of Justice. Who can stand against His Divination?

Peace is serving the world fruits of Truth, Justice, and Liberty for all humanity.

Peace is the river that quenches the thirst of all creatures.

To find peace, all must cast out follies.

To behold peace, all must chop down the wickedness in their imaginations.

To worship Peace, one must repent and reprove their deeds.

To understand Peace, one must seek Peace and fulfill Peace.

Peace leads us to the mountain of Justice where we all eat together in harmony, regardless of sex, religion, disability, or race.

On Heaven

Heaven is a kingdom where Peace reigns forever, and the Torch of Liberty burns forever, even in the silvery rain. Those who are loving are the flames of Beauty, and the storms cannot wipe out its glory.

Heaven is where sin and death do not exist, for the Father of Peace is the Warrior dressed in Glory who defeated all wickedness forever.

When you receive heaven, you will see that all things are free for our Creator is merciful and loves us.

Heaven is ageless and love surrounds us all.

If you seek faithfully Salvation and truly believe in the Heavenly Father, behold, the kingdom of Heaven is within you.

Heaven is the Promised Land flowing of milk and honey. Those who partake in this glory shall never thirst nor hunger for they are fulfilled.

Little children in heaven who were abused on earth are blessed forever.

Little children who were raped and murdered on earth have received the crown of eternal life and they shall never suffer again.

Heaven is the Spirit of Truth and Justice.

Heaven is the kingdom of eternal brotherhood without violence, greed, envy, jealousy, hate, deception, and ignorance.

Life is eternal for those who climb the invisible ladder to heaven. Though it is boundless, the beautiful ones never cease from seeking perfection.

Let your heart hold fast the ways of Truth so you may live to see heaven. For if you catch the feather of an angel, you shall turn into an angel when the shadow of Sin no longer binds you.

Without heaven, there is no life. Heaven is the Cradle that rocks the newborn spirits to eternal comfort and peace.

Let your spirit cast out all sins so you may live to inherit the treasures of heaven. For what child loves to play in the sandbox with shattered glass beneath the pebbles of sand?

All religions must unite under one Creator that created all glory in the heavens and the earth. If the earth cannot see this simplicity, the earth shall never see perfection.

Heaven is a place of universal glory. The righteous races of humanity are united in peace and liberty, for we are the spirits of Eternity.

Let your love stay in the light forever so you may see your Creator face to face.

On Eternal Life

Fire in which never dies, glory that shines forever. Legions of angels surround the throne of the Heavenly Father as wings of liberty dance and celebrate the glory of Life. Such is the Spirit of Peace. Such is the Kingdom of the Heavenly Father. Life is never short for the holy for they have eternal life.

To be strong is to build a temple of eternal life.

One that spends a lot of time serving souls of the earth is storing up treasures for eternal life.

Eternal life is the most glorious reward a spirit can receive.

Eternal life can only be found through faith in Life.

If one loves to commit sins, one will never see eternal life.

Stay in the light while you are in the light, and you shall see the Eternal light that gives life.

Eternal life can be described as a child seeking candy. The child does everything in its power to get the money to go to the candy store and buy its glory.

Even as one must drink the milk of life, one must drink the milk of death. Yet, one must drink the milk of eternal life to live again.

Why behold the anchor of eternal death when one can behold the Cloud of eternal life? Let all who love life never fade from doing good deeds, and those who love death, we can only hope you'll repent and reprove your deeds to spare your soul for eternity.

The farmers reap what is sowed, and the fruits of eternal life are given to their Master.

To those who defends Truth, Justice, and Liberty are the sons and daughters of Eternity, and we, the armies of Life, solute you.

Behold, thee who rewrites what is written in this book is not of the Heavenly Father and shall suffer the Wrath of Justice promised to those who worship Iniquity.

Made in the USA
Monee, IL
08 November 2026

67971946R00037